Peace Salad

100 TIPS

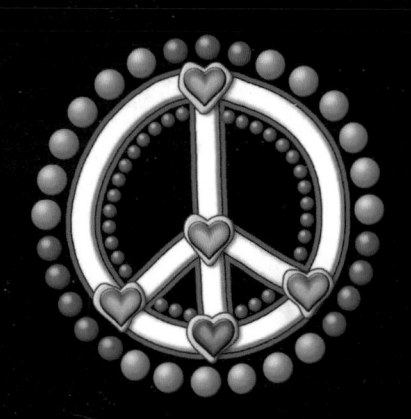

Sandy Henson Corso

Peace Salad

Peace Salad

(100 Tips to Inspire a Peaceful Life)

Sandy Henson Corso

PEACEFUL DAILY

Library of Congress Control Number: 2013901776

ISBN 978-0-9884926-0-8
EISBN 978-0-9884926-1-5

Cover and book design by Perseus Design
Peace Sign cover image © 2013 Tessla Queen

Published by Peaceful Daily
www.peacefuldaily.com

Printed in the United States of America.

First Edition

10 9 8 7 6 5 4 3 2 1

Dedicated to my beautiful family.

Gary, thank you for always
encouraging my soul to sing.

Topanga and Jaco, may you find
that which makes your soul sing.

Introduction

One day, we will experience global peace.

I would love to see this happen in my lifetime.

I believe that if we can find peace within ourselves, during our everyday lives, we can experience peace collectively and on a global scale.

My name is Sandy Corso, and I am the founder of Peaceful Daily, an online community that I created to inspire others to live their lives in a way that promotes compassion and connectivity.

Peaceful Daily supplies daily living tips to people around the world. Thousands of readers have sent emails describing how these tips changed their lives. I am so thankful for each and every reader.

Now, I bring you *Peace Salad*, a celebration of living with purpose and manifesting your dreams, while committing to well being! *Peace Salad* is a compilation of the most popular Peaceful Daily tips shared with our tribe of readers. Our tribe was founded on the mantra, "Think good. Eat whole. Walk far." Each tip in this book stems from one or more of these ideas.

Small and mighty, *Peace Salad* is filled with powerful messages. I carefully consolidated the most life-changing tips and knowledge into one simple book. After writing the book, I felt like I had put together just the right "manual" to help each of you find peace, happiness and wellness - no matter where you are in life.

Having weathered many storms, I speak from experience and apply each of these tips to my life. I often return to these thoughts as reminders, and I hope you will as well.

Whether trying to make the most of an ordinary day or overcome impossible challenges, you - and I - can discover and rediscover peace by applying the principles and philosophy inside these pages. I hope that in some way, *Peace Salad* brings peace to your life, too.

Enjoy!

Peace, Love and Happiness,
Sandy

100 TIPS

TIP 1

Contact each and every person
with whom you have experienced
any type of conflict
...no matter where they are on the planet.
Tell these people that you love them
and wish only the best for their lives.
Send each person love and forgiveness.
The hardest people to forgive
are the most important.
Forgive them anyway.
It is vital to your health!

TIP 2

Go barefoot as much as you can,
especially in nature!
Going barefoot
grounds our bodies to the earth's ionic charge
that extracts and expels negativity.
Walking without shoes on the ground
has been known to detoxify and calm.
If you love walking on the beach,
this tip may resonate with your spirit.

TIP 3

The best thing you can do for the world
is discover what makes your soul sing and
...GO DO IT!
The world needs
what you are meant to do.

TIP 4

When you wake up in the morning,
have a big glass of water
with fresh-squeezed lemon.
This will help your body detoxify after sleep,
when our bodies self cleanse and recalibrate.

TIP 5

Dry brush!
Your skin is like a third kidney.
Dry brushing removes dead skin cells
and improves blood and lymph circulation.

How to dry brush
Dry brush before you shower.
Beginning with your feet,
brush in sweeping motions,
moving toward the heart.
Brush your arms toward the heart,
and brush your neck and chest
with movement
toward the area underneath your arms.

TIP 6

Make sure you are breathing correctly!
Breathe in, slowly, through the nose,
allowing the lower belly to fill,
then, slowly, out of the mouth.

TIP 7

Drinking green juice once a day
can be life changing!
My favorite mixture is kale, celery,
ginger, lemon and cucumber.
All organic, of course.

TIP 8

Replace the way you refer
to the word "money"
with the word "energy,"
a life-affirming word.
Most people associate money
with negativity,
but if you change the word
…and your outlook…
the skies open up,
letting energy flow to you.

TIP 9

Hang a swing in your yard,
or even inside your home.
Swing often!
It will make you feel young and foolish.

TIP 10

Hug trees…
You can feel their healing energy.
Close your eyes,
and embrace.
Hugging trees is such a powerful thing…

TIP 11

Make sure all your body care products
(body wash, shampoo, conditioner, lotion)
never contain chemicals like parabens,
sodium lauryl sulfate and synthetic fragrances!

TIP 12

Yogis have been "tongue scraping"
for hundreds of years.
Ayurveda teaches
that tongue cleaning
helps with digestion **and** bacteria removal!

TIP 13

Only wear organic cotton underwear!
Cotton is considered
one of the most toxic textiles.
Underwear protects your private parts.
So, keep it organic.

TIP 14

A three-day juice fast
is known to detoxify
and regenerate.

TIP 15

Get 30 minutes of unprotected sun
every day.
It is the best source of vitamin D
– critical to overall health!

TIP 16

Be your own guru!

TIP 17

Cultivate your intuition,
just as you would your other studies
and interests.
Mastering your intuition
...the gateway to your dreams...
will bring you what you want in life.

TIP 18

Brush your teeth with baking soda
once a week.
Given all the claims
about baking soda's healing properties,
making this a ritual can't hurt.
Plus, your teeth will be whiter!

TIP 19

Try going vegetarian
for ethical and health reasons!

TIP 20

Cool word to know: Ahimsa.
Ahimsa is a Sanskrit word that means
to do no harm and avoid violence.

TIP 21

If you feel sad, blue or disconnected,
go for a 30-minute run.
You will feel much better
and reap heaps of health benefits.
Be sure to play your favorite music.
It'll make your run better and faster!

TIP 22

It has been scientifically proven
that thoughts are energy.
This truth means
you must be very diligent in your thinking.
Think and focus on the good stuff!

TIP 23

Give $100 to someone in need,
and do it anonymously!

TIP 24

Focus on the ways your job
helps make the world
a better place.

TIP 25

Chia seeds are a great vegetarian source
of omega 3s.

Chia seed pudding:
Mix three tablespoons of chia seeds
with one cup of almond milk.
Place in the fridge overnight.
Serve the next morning
with a dash of cinnamon!

TIP 26

Check your vitamin D and B12 levels regularly!

TIP 27

Did I mention the importance of laughter?
Look for any opportunity to laugh,
and laugh as much as possible.
Plan a visit with old friends
to laugh about old times.
It is the best medicine for me!

TIP 28

Fresh, raw fruits and vegetables
are the healthiest things
we can consume for our bodies.
Include daily servings of each in your diet.
Go raw for a week,
eating only raw fruits, vegetables, nuts and seeds.
Your body will thank you.

TIP 29

Seek reasons
to love
everything!

TIP 30

Stop trying to paddle upstream.
Let go of the oars.
Just flow
wherever destiny takes you.

TIP 31

Coconut oil
is a great facial moisturizer,
eye makeup remover
and hair gel.

TIP 32

Use Himalayan pink sea salt
instead of regular table salt.

TIP 33

Recycle when possible.
Composting is a great way to contribute
to our earth.

TIP 34

Create a vision board
that includes
everything
you want
in your life.

TIP 35

Examine all coincidences.
They are messages
and guidance
from the other side.

TIP 36

Take a yoga class
in extreme heat.
There is something magical about it!

TIP 37

For mind regeneration,
take a "clearing bath."

Clearing bath:
20 minutes in hot water
to which you add the following:
One pound of baking soda
Half a pound of sea salt
Five cups of apple cider vinegar
Light a candle,
and kiss your worries goodnight!

TIP 38

Get rid of your alarm clock.
If you are sleeping,
you need sleep.
Find a way to make it happen.

TIP 39

Sweat often.
Sweat helps release and clear out toxins.

TIP 40

Fast on water
for an entire day
(24 hours)!

TIP 41

Wherever you place your focus,
you will witness expansion.

TIP 42

Chew each mouthful of food
100 times.

TIP 43

Sleep with a cinnamon stick
under your pillow.
A cinnamon stick is known for the ability
to capture lingering negative energy
that may come out of your dreams!

TIP 44

Every day,
do something that scares you.

TIP 45

Use diluted peppermint castile soap
to clean almost anything on you
or in your house,
including your body, teeth, hair,
dirty shoes, kids' feet, dishes, produce,
floors, countertops, showers, clothes
…even your dog!

TIP 46

When hosting a party,
be sure to pass around a gratitude napkin!
All you need is a blank cloth napkin
and permanent marker.
Let everyone write about their blessings
on the gratitude napkin,
which you will cherish for years to come.

TIP 47

Tantric love!
Google it!

TIP 48

Flow doesn't happen
with separation.
Flow happens with connection!

TIP 49

I believe our body
has the ability
to heal itself
without drugs.
If you believe you can heal,
you probably will.

TIP 50

We are all concerned
with being compassionate
toward less fortunate people in the world.
In the same way,
we should be mindful of self compassion
and the crying child inside of each one of us.
Take time for self-compassion.

TIP 51

When possible, try to buy the following organic:
apples, celery, bell peppers, peaches,
strawberries, nectarines, grapes, spinach,
lettuce, cucumbers, blueberries and potatoes.

Also, to reduce the GMOs in your diet,
consider buying organic corn and soy.

TIP 52

An aloe vera plant
is the best addition to any first aid kit.
This miracle plant has been used
for thousands of years
to remedy many ills!

TIP 53

Give up your need to impress others!
Focus on impressing
yourself.

TIP 54

Wear your hair in pigtails.
It will make you look
10 years younger.

TIP 55

Five minutes of meditation
will enhance your life
…more than most things.

TIP 56

Drink lots of water.
Keep drinking water
until your pee is clear,
not yellow.

TIP 57

Music can transform your life.
I believe it is the energy
that connects us
with the heavens…

TIP 58

Jumping on a mini-trampoline (rebounding)
is one of the best exercises
for your body and mind,
mainly because
it gets your lymphatic system moving
and helps boost your immune system!

TIP 59

If you had 10 million dollars in the bank,
what would you do?
Write down your ideas,
and start executing!

TIP 60

Massage may seem like a luxury!
It is much more than a luxury.
The power of touch
is an important step
toward health and healing!

TIP 61

Tap on your meridian points
while focusing and repeating
positive affirmations.

Meridian Tapping:
With your fingers,
start tapping the side of your hand.
Then, move to the area
of your forehead
just above the space
where your eyebrows begin,
and then to each side of your head
(your temples),
under your eyes, under your nose,
on your chin, on your collarbone,
under your arms
and, finally, the top of your head.

TIP 62

The best present you can give yourself
is the gift of forgiveness.
First, forgive yourself
...and then everyone else!

TIP 63

Now that you are a vegetarian,
try going vegan!
Eliminate all animal products
from your diet and life.
Yes - this includes pizza
and your favorite leather shoes!

TIP 64

When you get a boo-boo,
give yourself a kiss
and imagine the presence
of a healing white light!
This is a great tip to teach kids.

TIP 65

Another cool word to know: Ubuntu.
Ubuntu refers to interconnection
and the importance of a group working together
for the greater good.

TIP 66

Give more
in service
than you take in money.

TIP 67

It is rumored you need
12 hugs a day.
How many hugs have you had today?

TIP 68

Act as if it already is.

TIP 69

Learn to make your own salad dressing.
This is an important talent
that ensures you will eat lots of salad.

TIP 70

Three to four a.m. is a mystical time.
If you wake up
during these early and sacred morning hours,
enjoy the time.
This is when many people
produce their most creative work!

TIP 71

Host a vegan potluck!
Inspire your friends and family
with healthy eating
by getting everyone involved.
These get-togethers are amazingly popular
and lots of fun!

TIP 72

Be willing to tell your lover
what you want.

TIP 73

Sleep with an open window.
While you are sleeping,
it is so important to have fresh air circulating
throughout the room.
My grandmother, who lived to be 96,
read *Prevention Magazine*,
never took medication (not even aspirin)
and always slept with her bedroom window open
…just a crack…
even in freezing temperatures.

TIP 74

Long hair is believed to make you more intuitive!
A natural extension of the nervous system,
hair serves as a direct link to our brain
and emits energy into the environment.

TIP 75

Turmeric:
Put it on everything!

TIP 76

Talk more about what is
possible,
rather than what actually is.

TIP 77

Wabi Sabi is the art of imperfection.
Real beauty lives here.

TIP 78

Clutter:
Get rid of it!

TIP 79

What are you willing to do for free?
Observe closely.
This is where you will find
the key to your success.

TIP 80

Write a love letter
to your body.

TIP 81

Morning intentions have proven to be
an important habit!
As soon as my eyes open in the morning,
I start to visualize
how my day will go.
I visualize myself
eating beautiful colorful fruits
and veggies.
I see myself at the gym
covered in sweat.
I see my family laughing
and being happy.
I see myself
completing household chores
with a smile.
**I see myself joyful
that I am
getting things done.**

TIP 82

Cultivate compassion
for all living things.

TIP 83

Dream
even bigger
than your greatest imaginings.

TIP 84

Kindness rules.
Always look for ways to be a kind human being.

TIP 85

There is an Indian prophecy
about Rainbow Warriors,
a group of people
that will someday inhabit the earth
and save all living things from environmental crisis.
If you are reading this book,
you are probably a Rainbow Warrior!

TIP 86

If you eat meat and dairy,
please consider organic,
grass fed
and cage free varieties.

TIP 87

Conflicts with loved ones can be so trying!
I have found that when dealing
with these situations,
the best thing to do
(with all your might)
is focus on the good qualities of that person.
Then, the bad qualities fade away!

TIP 88

Throw out your umbrella,
and walk in the rain.
Feel the rain falling
on your face!

TIP 89

Always carry a reusable water bottle.
Bottled water is bad for the planet!

TIP 90

Pets:
Have as many as you can.
They bring me so much peace.

TIP 91

Quinoa is a complete protein
and considered a perfect grain,
meaning it contains
all eight essential amino acids.

TIP 92

Always use natural deodorants.
Did you know that a lime makes a great deodorant?
Cut and place a lime in the fridge.
Use under your arms
every morning.
Remember to label the lime.

TIP 93

Prayers work.

TIP 94

Find gratitude in the smallest
and most insignificant
things.

TIP 95

You have not lived
until you have experienced
a Kundalini Awakening.

TIP 96

Save the bees.

TIP 97

When you implement the following words,
change really happens…
*There is no way to make
or even inspire others
to be happy
until you make yourself happy
first.*

TIP 98

Hand selected friends can be as important
as blood family.

TIP 99

Remove all toxic cleaning supplies from your home.
Never buy these items again,
and replace
with the most natural products you can find.
No matter what your mother says,
it is *never good* to have bleach in the house!

TIP 100

Anger bleeds the heart,
and hatred dehydrates the spirit!
Love and peace heal all!
In every situation, turn to love!

Gratitude for you!

About the Author

SANDY HENSON CORSO is the founder of Peaceful Daily. Her passion is the holistic world, and her voice is a reflection of that passion. Sandy's engaged and active audience shares in her adventures and quest to live a more peaceful life. She brings a fresh, innovative perspective to all aspects of living the holistic way.

Peaceful Daily is the manifestation of Sandy's desire to create a community founded on principles of compassion, well being, and taking action to make the world a better place.

Sandy lives in Connecticut with her husband, two young children (Topanga and Jaco), a dog named Bosco and a cat named Emily Google.

If you dig this book, you can follow Sandy here:

Peaceful Daily
www.peacefuldaily.com

The Huffington Post
www.huffingtonpost.com/sandy-henson-corso

What are you grateful for?

CPSIA information can be obtained at www.ICGtesting.com
Printed in the USA
BVOW031132040413

317312BV00002B/28/P